Whole Food Easy to Use Guide for Beginners

Incorporating Whole Foods into Your Lifestyle

By

Mannix Latharn

Copyright@2023

Table of Contents

CHAPTER 1

Introduction

In the contemporary landscape of nutrition and wellness, the emphasis on whole foods has gained substantial traction. This introduction seeks to unravel the myriad benefits that whole foods offer, positioning them as a cornerstone for promoting holistic health and well-being.

1.1 Benefits of Whole Foods

Whole foods, in their unadulterated and unprocessed state, constitute a treasure trove of essential nutrients that are integral to sustaining a healthy lifestyle. Herein lies a compendium of benefits that underscores the significance of incorporating whole foods into one's diet.

Nutrient Density: Whole foods, such as fruits, vegetables, whole grains, and lean proteins, are rich in essential vitamins, minerals, fiber, and antioxidants. Unlike processed foods that often contain empty calories and additives, whole foods boast unparalleled nutrient density. This means that even in moderate quantities, they provide a wealth of nutrients crucial for various physiological functions, from cellular repair to immune system support.

Disease Prevention: The consumption of whole foods has been linked to a reduced risk of chronic diseases, including heart disease, diabetes, and certain cancers. The abundance of antioxidants and phytochemicals in fruits and vegetables, for example, contributes to combating oxidative stress and inflammation, two key factors implicated in the development of chronic illnesses.

Weight Management: In the pursuit of maintaining a healthy weight, the role of whole foods is pivotal. These foods are often rich in fiber, which promotes satiety and helps regulate appetite. Moreover, the complex carbohydrates found in whole grains release energy gradually, providing a sustained feeling of fullness and preventing the rapid spikes and crashes in blood sugar associated with refined carbohydrates.

Digestive Health: The fiber content in whole foods is instrumental in fostering a healthy digestive system. Fiber adds bulk to the diet, aiding in regular bowel movements and preventing constipation. Additionally, it supports the growth of beneficial gut bacteria, contributing to a balanced and thriving microbiome, which has been increasingly recognized as crucial for overall health.

Energy and Vitality: Whole foods are a source of sustained energy, steering clear of the temporary boosts followed by energy slumps associated with processed foods. The vitamins and minerals present in whole foods play a crucial role in energy metabolism, ensuring that the body efficiently converts nutrients into usable energy, promoting vitality and overall well-being.

Mental Health and Cognitive Function: Emerging research suggests a strong connection between diet and mental health. Whole foods, rich in omega-3 fatty acids, antioxidants, and vitamins, have been associated with a lower risk of depression and cognitive decline. Nourishing the body with a spectrum of nutrients contributes to optimal brain function, supporting memory, focus, and overall cognitive performance.

Environmental Sustainability: Beyond personal health, the benefits of whole foods extend to the broader environment. Embracing a diet centered on whole, plant-based foods often has a lower environmental impact, requiring fewer resources and producing fewer greenhouse gas emissions compared to the production of processed and animal-based foods. Making conscious choices in food consumption aligns not only with individual health goals but also with global sustainability efforts.

The benefits of whole foods are multifaceted, encompassing physical health, disease prevention, mental well-being, and ecological sustainability. As we delve into the nuances of this guide, the journey toward embracing whole foods emerges not only as a personal quest for health but also as a conscientious choice with far-reaching implications for the individual and the planet.

CHAPTER 2

Understanding Whole Foods

In the journey towards a healthier lifestyle, understanding the essence of whole foods is fundamental.

2.1 Definition of Whole Foods

Whole foods refer to natural, unprocessed, and unrefined foods that are as close to their original state as possible. These foods are minimally altered, preserving their inherent nutritional content. Whole foods encompass a broad spectrum of fresh, uncooked fruits and vegetables, whole grains, lean proteins, nuts, seeds, and legumes. The key principle is to consume foods that are in or close to their natural form, avoiding the additives, preservatives, and refining processes often associated with processed counterparts.

The emphasis on whole foods is rooted in the belief that their natural state preserves the synergy of nutrients and compounds that work together to optimize health. By consuming foods in their entirety, individuals harness the collective benefits of vitamins, minerals, antioxidants, fiber, and other bioactive substances that contribute to overall well-being.

2.2 Nutritional Value

The nutritional value of whole foods is unparalleled, providing a comprehensive array of essential nutrients necessary for the body's optimal functioning. These foods are rich in vitamins and minerals, which are crucial for various physiological processes, including energy metabolism, immune function, and bone health.

Moreover, whole foods are abundant sources of dietary fiber, promoting digestive health and aiding in weight management. The fiber content contributes to a feeling of fullness, regulating appetite and preventing overeating. Additionally, whole foods often contain healthy fats, such as omega-3 fatty acids found in fatty fish and nuts, which support cardiovascular health and cognitive function.

The presence of antioxidants in many whole foods further enhances their nutritional profile. Antioxidants combat oxidative stress, a process implicated in aging and the development of chronic diseases. By neutralizing free radicals, these compounds contribute to cellular health and may reduce the risk of conditions like heart disease and certain cancers.

2.3 Types of Whole Foods

Whole foods encompass a diverse range of categories, each offering unique nutritional benefits. Understanding the types of whole foods allows individuals to create a balanced and varied diet. The primary categories include:

- **Fruits and Vegetables:** Rich in vitamins, minerals, fiber, and antioxidants, fruits and vegetables form the foundation of a whole-foods-based diet. Varieties of colors and types ensure a broad spectrum of nutrients.

- **Whole Grains:** Whole grains, such as brown rice, quinoa, and oats, retain the bran, germ, and endosperm, providing fiber, vitamins, and minerals. They are essential for sustained energy and digestive health.

- **Lean Proteins:** Sources like poultry, fish, tofu, legumes, and beans offer high-quality proteins without the added saturated fats often present in processed meats.

- **Nuts and Seeds:** Packed with healthy fats, protein, and various nutrients, nuts and seeds make for excellent snacks and additions to meals, supporting heart health and providing essential micronutrients.

- **Dairy and Alternatives:** Unprocessed dairy products and plant-based alternatives like almond or soy milk provide calcium, vitamin D, and other nutrients crucial for bone health.

- **Legumes:** Beans, lentils, and chickpeas are rich in protein, fiber, and various vitamins, serving as a versatile and nutritious component of a whole-foods diet.

Incorporating a variety of these whole foods into daily meals, individuals can create a nutrient-dense and well-balanced diet that promotes overall health and vitality. Understanding the nutritional value and diversity within each category empowers individuals to make informed choices, fostering a holistic approach to nutrition.

CHAPTER 3

Getting Started with Whole Foods

Embarking on a journey toward embracing whole foods is a transformative step towards better health and well-being.

3.1 Importance of Transitioning

The shift from a conventional diet to one centered around whole foods is a significant and positive change that can yield numerous health benefits. Transitioning to whole foods is essential for several reasons:

- **Nutrient Density:** Whole foods are rich in essential nutrients, offering a potent mix of vitamins, minerals, fiber, and antioxidants. This nutrient density ensures that the body receives the necessary building blocks for optimal functioning, promoting overall health and vitality.

- **Disease Prevention:** Numerous studies suggest that a diet focused on whole foods can reduce the risk of chronic diseases such as heart disease, diabetes, and certain cancers. The natural compounds found in whole foods, coupled with their anti-inflammatory properties, contribute to a lower risk of developing these conditions.

- **Weight Management:** Whole foods, particularly those high in fiber, contribute to a feeling of fullness and satiety. This can aid in weight management by preventing overeating and promoting a balanced caloric intake.

- **Stable Energy Levels:** Unlike the energy spikes and crashes associated with processed foods, whole foods provide sustained energy. The complex carbohydrates found in whole grains, coupled with the nutrients in fruits and vegetables, support stable blood sugar levels, preventing fatigue and promoting sustained vitality.

- **Digestive Health:** The fiber content in whole foods supports

a healthy digestive system.
Fiber adds bulk to the diet, aids
in regular bowel movements,
and fosters a balanced gut
microbiome, contributing to
optimal digestive function.

- **Mental Well-being:** Emerging
research suggests a link
between diet and mental health.
Whole foods, rich in omega-3
fatty acids, antioxidants, and
vitamins, have been associated
with a lower risk of depression
and cognitive decline,
promoting overall mental well-
being.

3.2 Planning Your Whole Food Journey

A successful transition to a whole-
foods-based diet requires thoughtful

planning. Consider the following steps to guide your journey:

- **Educate Yourself:** Learn about the benefits of whole foods, understand different food categories, and familiarize yourself with nutrient-rich options. Knowledge forms the foundation for making informed choices.

- **Assess Your Current Diet:** Take stock of your current eating habits. Identify processed and refined foods that can be gradually replaced with whole alternatives. Recognize patterns, preferences, and potential challenges.

- **Gradual Changes:** Instead of an abrupt overhaul, introduce whole foods gradually. Start by incorporating more fruits, vegetables, and whole grains into your meals. Experiment with new recipes and flavors to make the transition enjoyable.

- **Meal Planning:** Plan your meals in advance to ensure a balanced intake of nutrients. Create shopping lists that prioritize whole, unprocessed foods. This helps in avoiding impulse purchases of processed items.

- **Experiment with Cooking:** Embrace the joy of cooking with whole ingredients. Experimenting with recipes not only enhances your culinary skills but also makes the transition to whole foods more exciting and sustainable.

3.3 Setting Realistic Goals

Setting realistic and achievable goals is crucial for long-term success in adopting a whole-foods-based lifestyle. Consider the following when establishing your goals:

- **Start Small:** Begin with achievable goals that align with your current lifestyle. Whether it's incorporating one additional serving of vegetables per day or swapping a processed snack for a whole-food alternative, small changes build momentum.

- **Be Specific:** Define clear and specific goals. Rather than a vague aim to "eat healthier," set targets like "consume at least three servings of vegetables daily" or "replace one processed snack with a piece of fresh fruit."

- **Gradual Progression:** Allow for a gradual progression towards a predominantly whole-foods diet. This approach is more sustainable and reduces the likelihood of feeling overwhelmed.

- **Track Your Progress:** Keep a journal or use apps to track your progress. Celebrate achievements, reflect on challenges, and adjust goals accordingly. Tracking provides valuable insights into your evolving relationship with whole foods.

- **Seek Support:** Share your goals with friends, family, or join communities focused on whole-food living. Having a support system can provide encouragement, share experiences, and offer valuable tips for overcoming challenges.

The importance of transitioning to a whole-foods-based diet cannot be overstated. By understanding the benefits, planning your journey, and setting realistic goals, you pave the way for a sustainable and transformative shift towards a healthier and more vibrant lifestyle.

CHAPTER 4

Identifying Whole Foods

Recognizing and selecting whole foods is a pivotal aspect of transitioning to a healthier diet.

4.1 Grocery Shopping Tips

Efficient grocery shopping is a key component of adopting a whole-foods-based diet. Consider these tips to navigate the aisles effectively:

- **Shop the Perimeter:** Whole foods, such as fresh produce, lean proteins, dairy, and whole grains, are often situated around the perimeter of the grocery store. Focus on these areas to prioritize nutrient-dense options.

- **Create a List:** Plan your meals and create a shopping list before heading to the store. This helps you stay focused on whole, unprocessed ingredients and reduces the likelihood of impulse purchases.

- **Buy Seasonal Produce:** Seasonal fruits and vegetables are not only fresher but also more affordable. Check for local produce, as it often aligns with the seasons and supports regional agriculture.

- **Explore Bulk Sections:** Many grocery stores have bulk sections offering grains, nuts, seeds, and legumes. Buying in bulk can be cost-effective and minimizes packaging waste.

- **Read Ingredient Lists:** Pay attention to the ingredients listed on packaged foods. Whole foods should have minimal, recognizable ingredients. Avoid products with long lists of additives, preservatives, and artificial substances.

- **Choose Whole Grains:** Opt for whole grains like brown rice, quinoa, and oats instead of refined grains. Whole grains retain their fiber and nutrients, offering a more wholesome option.

- **Prioritize Fresh and Minimally Processed Options:** Select fresh foods over processed alternatives. For example, choose whole fruits instead of fruit juices or whole grains instead of refined flour products.

- **Be Mindful of Labels:** Understand food labels and certifications. Look for terms like "organic," "non-GMO," and "grass-fed" to ensure the quality of the product.

4.2 Reading Food Labels

Navigating food labels is crucial for identifying whole foods and making informed choices. Consider the following tips when reading labels:

- **Check the Ingredient List:** The ingredient list provides insight into the composition of the product. Whole foods should have short ingredient lists with items you recognize as real food.

- **Look for Whole Grains:** When selecting grain products, ensure that the word "whole" precedes the grain (e.g., whole wheat, whole oats). This indicates that the product contains the entire grain kernel.

- **Watch for Additives:** Be cautious of products with excessive additives, preservatives, and artificial colors. Opt for products with minimal processing and a focus on natural ingredients.

- **Mind Serving Sizes:** Pay attention to serving sizes to accurately assess nutritional content. Some products may appear healthy at first glance but may have small serving sizes that can be misleading.

- **Understand Nutrient Claims:** Phrases like "low-fat," "high-fiber," or "sugar-free" can sometimes be misleading. Always check the nutritional information to get a comprehensive view of the product.

4.3 Common Whole Food Choices

Understanding the variety of whole foods available is essential for diversifying your diet. Here are some common whole food choices to consider:

- **Fruits:** Apples, berries, oranges, bananas, and melons.

- **Vegetables:** Leafy greens, broccoli, carrots, bell peppers, and sweet potatoes.

- **Whole Grains:** Brown rice, quinoa, oats, barley, and whole wheat products.

- **Lean Proteins:** Chicken, turkey, fish, tofu, legumes, and eggs.

- **Nuts and Seeds:** Almonds, walnuts, chia seeds, flaxseeds, and sunflower seeds.

- **Dairy and Alternatives:** Greek yogurt, milk, cheese, and plant-based alternatives like almond or soy milk.

- **Legumes:** Lentils, chickpeas, black beans, and kidney beans.

Incorporating these common whole foods into your shopping list and meals, you ensure a diverse and nutrient-rich diet that aligns with the principles of whole-food living. These choices form the foundation of a healthful and satisfying culinary experience.

CHAPTER 5

Easy whole Food Recipes for Beginners

Embracing a whole-foods-based lifestyle is made more accessible with simple and delicious recipes. This section provides beginner-friendly options for breakfast and lunch, ensuring a flavorful and nutritious start to your day and a satisfying midday meal.

5.1 Breakfast Options

1. Overnight Oats:

- **Ingredients:**

- 1/2 cup rolled oats

- 1/2 cup Greek yogurt

- 1/2 cup milk (dairy or plant-based)

- 1 tablespoon chia seeds

- 1/2 teaspoon vanilla extract

- Fresh fruits (berries, banana slices) for topping

- Nuts or seeds for crunch (e.g., almonds, walnuts)

- **Instructions:**

1. In a jar, combine oats, yogurt, milk, chia seeds, and vanilla extract.

2. Stir well, cover, and refrigerate overnight.

3. In the morning, give it a good stir, top with fresh fruits and nuts,

and enjoy a quick and nutritious breakfast.

2. Avocado Toast:

- **Ingredients:**

- 1 slice whole-grain bread

- 1/2 ripe avocado

- Cherry tomatoes, sliced

- Salt and pepper to taste

- Optional toppings: poached egg, red pepper flakes, or feta cheese

- **Instructions:**

1. Toast the whole-grain bread slice.

2. Mash the ripe avocado and spread it over the toast.

3. Top with sliced cherry tomatoes, salt, and pepper.

4. Customize with optional toppings based on your preferences.

3. Greek Yogurt Parfait:

- **Ingredients:**

- 1 cup Greek yogurt

- Granola

- Mixed berries (blueberries, strawberries)

- Honey or maple syrup for drizzling

- **Instructions:**

1. In a glass or bowl, layer Greek yogurt, granola, and mixed berries.

2. Repeat the layers.

3. Drizzle honey or maple syrup on top.

4. Enjoy a delicious and protein-packed parfait.

5.2 Lunch Ideas

1. Quinoa Salad:

- **Ingredients:**

- 1 cup cooked quinoa

- Cherry tomatoes, halved

- Cucumber, diced

- Red bell pepper, chopped

- Feta cheese, crumbled

- Fresh parsley, chopped

- Olive oil and lemon juice dressing

- **Instructions:**

1. In a bowl, combine cooked quinoa, cherry tomatoes, cucumber, red bell pepper, feta cheese, and fresh parsley.

2. Drizzle with olive oil and lemon juice, toss well, and serve as a refreshing quinoa salad.

2. Chickpea Wrap:

- **Ingredients:**

- Whole-grain wrap

- 1 cup canned chickpeas, drained and rinsed

- Cherry tomatoes, sliced

- Cucumber, julienned

- Spinach leaves

- Hummus for spreading

- **Instructions:**

1. In a bowl, mash chickpeas with a fork.

2. Spread hummus on the whole-grain wrap.

3. Add mashed chickpeas, cherry tomatoes, cucumber, and spinach.

4. Wrap it up and enjoy a satisfying and protein-packed lunch.

3. Vegetable Stir-Fry:

- **Ingredients:**

- Mixed vegetables (broccoli, bell peppers, carrots, snap peas)

- Tofu or chicken breast, cubed

- Soy sauce

- Garlic, minced

- Ginger, grated

- Brown rice (cooked)

- **Instructions:**

  1. In a pan, stir-fry tofu or chicken until cooked.

  2. Add mixed vegetables, garlic, and ginger. Cook until vegetables are tender-crisp.

  3. Drizzle with soy sauce and toss.

  4. Serve over cooked brown rice for a quick and wholesome stir-fry.

These easy and delicious recipes are perfect for beginners looking to incorporate whole foods into their breakfast and lunch routines. They not only provide essential nutrients but also make the transition to a whole-foods-based diet enjoyable and sustainable.

5.3 Dinner Recipes

1. Baked Salmon with Roasted Vegetables:

- **Ingredients:**

- Salmon fillets

- Asparagus spears

- Cherry tomatoes

- Red onion, sliced

- Olive oil

- Lemon juice

- Garlic, minced

- Fresh herbs (such as dill or parsley)

- Salt and pepper

- **Instructions:**

1. Preheat the oven to 400°F (200°C).

2. Place salmon fillets on a baking sheet and surround them with asparagus, cherry tomatoes, and sliced red onion.

3. In a bowl, mix olive oil, lemon juice, minced garlic, fresh herbs, salt, and pepper. Drizzle this mixture over the salmon and vegetables.

4. Bake for 15-20 minutes or until the salmon is cooked through and the vegetables are roasted.

2. Quinoa and Vegetable Stir-Fry:

- **Ingredients:**

- Cooked quinoa

- Mixed vegetables (broccoli, bell peppers, carrots, snap peas)

- Tofu or shrimp

- Soy sauce

- Sesame oil

- Ginger, grated

- Garlic, minced

- Green onions, chopped

- **Instructions:**

1. In a wok or pan, stir-fry tofu or shrimp until cooked.

2. Add mixed vegetables, grated ginger, and minced garlic. Cook until vegetables are tender-crisp.

3. Add cooked quinoa, soy sauce, and a drizzle of sesame oil. Toss until well combined.

4. Garnish with chopped green onions and serve.

3. Sweet Potato and Chickpea Curry:

- **Ingredients:**

- Sweet potatoes, diced

- Chickpeas (canned, drained and rinsed)

- Coconut milk

- Curry paste

- Onion, diced

- Garlic, minced

- Spinach leaves

- Basmati rice (cooked)

- **Instructions:**

1. In a pot, sauté diced onions and garlic until softened.

2. Add sweet potatoes, chickpeas, coconut milk, and curry paste. Simmer until sweet potatoes are tender.

3. Stir in fresh spinach until wilted.

4. Serve over cooked basmati rice for a hearty and flavorful curry.

5.4 Snack Suggestions

1. Greek Yogurt and Berry Bowl:

- **Ingredients:**

- Greek yogurt

- Mixed berries (blueberries, strawberries, raspberries)

- Honey or maple syrup

- Granola

- **Instructions:**

  1. In a bowl, layer Greek yogurt, mixed berries, and granola.

  2. Drizzle with honey or maple syrup for sweetness.

  3. Enjoy a satisfying and protein-packed snack.

2. Hummus and Vegetable Sticks:

- **Ingredients:**

- Hummus (store-bought or homemade)

- Carrot sticks

- Cucumber slices

- Bell pepper strips

- **Instructions:**

  1. Arrange vegetable sticks on a plate.

  2. Dip the sticks into hummus for a crunchy and nutritious snack.

3. Almond Butter and Banana Slices:

- **Ingredients:**

- Almond butter (or any nut butter)

- Banana, sliced

- Whole-grain rice cakes or whole wheat crackers

- **Instructions:**

1. Spread almond butter on rice cakes or crackers.

2. Top with banana slices for a quick and energy-boosting snack.

These dinner recipes and snack suggestions are not only delicious but also align with the principles of a whole-foods-based diet. They incorporate a variety of nutrient-dense ingredients to ensure you enjoy flavorful and satisfying meals throughout the day.

CHAPTER 6

Meal Planning and Prepping

Efficient meal planning and prepping are instrumental in maintaining a whole-foods-based lifestyle.

6.1 Creating a Whole Food Meal Plan

Creating a thoughtful meal plan ensures a balanced intake of nutrients and simplifies your grocery shopping and cooking process. Here's a guide to crafting a whole food meal plan:

- **Assess Nutritional Needs:** Consider your dietary preferences, nutritional requirements, and any specific health goals. Ensure your meal plan includes a variety of fruits, vegetables, whole grains, lean proteins, and healthy fats.

- **Plan Balanced Meals:** Design meals that incorporate a mix of macronutrients (carbohydrates, proteins, and fats) and a variety of colors and textures. Aim for a rainbow of fruits and vegetables to maximize nutritional diversity.

- **Rotate Proteins:** Include a variety of protein sources such as lean meats, poultry, fish, tofu, legumes, and dairy. Rotate protein options throughout the week to ensure a well-rounded intake of essential amino acids.

- **Incorporate Whole Grains:** Opt for whole grains like brown rice, quinoa, barley, and oats to provide sustained energy and a rich source of fiber.

- **Embrace Seasonal Produce:** Plan meals based on seasonal fruits and vegetables. Not only does this support local agriculture, but it also ensures fresher and more flavorful ingredients.

- **Prepare Snacks:** Include wholesome snacks like fresh fruit, vegetable sticks with hummus, or a handful of nuts to curb between-meal hunger and provide additional nutrients.

- **Keep Hydration in Mind:** Include water, herbal teas, and infused water in your meal plan. Staying hydrated is essential for overall health.

- **Be Flexible:** Allow room for flexibility in your meal plan. Life can be unpredictable, and having a flexible approach makes it easier to adapt to changing circumstances.

6.2 Batch Cooking Tips

Batch cooking is a time-saving strategy that involves preparing larger quantities of food to have ready-made meals throughout the week. Here are tips for successful batch cooking:

- **Choose Batch-Friendly Recipes:** Opt for recipes that can be easily scaled up and maintain their quality after being reheated. Soups, stews, casseroles, and grain bowls are excellent choices for batch cooking.

- **Invest in Storage Containers:** Use a variety of containers for storing batch-cooked meals. Consider glass or BPA-free plastic containers that are microwave-safe and stackable.

- **Label and Date:** Label each container with the contents and date of preparation to keep track of freshness. Use a rotation system, placing newer batches at the back of the fridge or freezer.

- **Portion Control:** Divide batch-cooked meals into individual or family-sized portions before storing. This makes it easy to grab a pre-portioned meal for reheating.

- **Utilize Freezer-Friendly Foods:** Some foods freeze better than others. Soups, stews, cooked grains, and casseroles often maintain their quality after freezing. Freeze in portioned containers for convenient use.

- **Plan a Batch Cooking Day:** Dedicate a specific day of the week to batch cooking. This can streamline your weekly routine and ensure you always have nutritious options on hand.

6.3 Storing Whole Foods

Proper storage helps maintain the freshness and quality of whole foods. Follow these guidelines for storing various whole foods:

- **Fruits and Vegetables:**

  - Store fruits and vegetables separately to prevent ethylene-producing fruits from accelerating ripening in others.

  - Keep fruits and vegetables in the crisper drawer of the refrigerator.

  - Some items, like tomatoes, avocados, and bananas, can be stored at room temperature until ripe.

- **Whole Grains:**

  - Store whole grains in airtight containers to prevent moisture and pests.

  - Keep grains in a cool, dark place to maintain freshness.

- **Lean Proteins:**

  - Refrigerate or freeze lean proteins based on their freshness and when they will be used.

  - Divide larger portions into smaller ones for more efficient storage.

- **Nuts and Seeds:**

- Store nuts and seeds in airtight containers in a cool, dark place or the refrigerator to prevent rancidity.

    - Consider buying in smaller quantities to ensure freshness.

- **Dairy and Alternatives:**

    - Keep dairy products and plant-based alternatives in the refrigerator.

    - Check expiration dates and consume within the recommended timeframe.

- **Batch-Cooked Meals:**

    - Refrigerate or freeze batch-cooked meals promptly after preparation.

- Use airtight containers or freezer-safe bags to prevent freezer burn.

These meal planning, batch cooking, and storage tips into your routine, you can streamline the process of maintaining a whole-foods-based lifestyle, making it more convenient and sustainable in the long run.

CHAPTER 7

Overcoming Challenges

Adopting a whole-foods-based lifestyle comes with its set of challenges.

7.1 Dealing with Cravings

Cravings for processed or unhealthy foods can pose a challenge when transitioning to a whole-foods diet. Here are strategies to manage and overcome cravings:

- **Understand the Root Cause:**

  - Reflect on the source of your cravings. Is it emotional, habit-driven, or tied to specific situations? Understanding the root cause helps address cravings more effectively.

- **Stay Hydrated:**

  - Dehydration can sometimes be mistaken for hunger. Ensure you stay adequately hydrated throughout the day, as this may help curb unnecessary cravings.

- **Include Satisfying Whole Foods:**

  - Integrate satisfying whole foods into your meals to prevent feelings of deprivation. Incorporate a variety of flavors, textures, and nutrient-dense options.

- **Plan Healthy Alternatives:**

  - Have nutritious alternatives ready for when cravings strike. For example, keep a bowl of fresh fruit, a handful of nuts, or vegetable sticks with hummus on hand.

- **Mindful Eating Practices:**

  - Practice mindful eating by savoring each bite and paying attention to hunger and fullness cues. This can help you become more attuned to your body's needs.

- **Allow Occasional Treats:**

- It's okay to indulge in treats occasionally. Allow yourself small portions of your favorite treats to satisfy cravings without derailing your overall healthy eating plan.

7.2 Social and Lifestyle Considerations

Social events and lifestyle factors can sometimes pose challenges to maintaining a whole-foods-based diet. Here's how to navigate such situations:

- **Communicate Your Preferences:**

  - Communicate your dietary preferences to

friends and family. Let them know about your commitment to a whole-foods lifestyle so that they can offer support.

- **Bring Your Own Dish:**

    - If attending a social gathering or event, consider bringing a whole-foods-based dish to share. This ensures you have a nutritious option available.

- **Choose Wisely at Restaurants:**

    - When dining out, opt for restaurants that offer whole-foods-based options. Check menus in advance and make

choices that align with
your dietary goals.

- **Be Prepared:**

  - Keep healthy snacks on
    hand for times when
    whole-foods options may
    be limited. Having a
    piece of fruit, a small bag
    of nuts, or a snack bar
    can prevent impulsive
    choices.

- **Focus on the Experience:**

  - Shift the focus of social
    events from the food to
    the experience. Engage
    in conversations,
    activities, and enjoy the
    company of others rather
    than solely focusing on
    the menu.

7.3 Troubleshooting Common Issues

Addressing common issues that may arise during the transition to a whole-foods-based lifestyle is essential for long-term success. Here are strategies to troubleshoot challenges:

- **Time Constraints:**

  - Plan and prioritize meal prep during times that fit your schedule. Batch cooking on weekends or preparing meals in advance can save time during busy weekdays.

- **Budgetary Constraints:**

  - Whole foods can sometimes be perceived as more expensive. Focus on cost-effective options like seasonal produce, buying in bulk, and planning meals to minimize food waste.

- **Limited Culinary Skills:**

  - Build your culinary skills gradually. Start with simple recipes and gradually experiment with new techniques and ingredients. Cooking classes or online tutorials can be helpful.

- **Taste Preferences:**

  - Experiment with various whole foods and cooking methods to discover flavors and textures you enjoy. Trying new recipes can be an exciting way to find

whole foods that align
with your taste
preferences.

- **Digestive Issues:**

  - If you experience
    digestive discomfort
    when incorporating more
    whole foods, introduce
    them gradually. High-
    fiber foods, in particular,
    may require an
    adjustment period for
    your digestive system.

- **Lack of Variety:**

  - Ensure variety in your
    meals by exploring
    different whole foods,
    herbs, and spices. Rotate
    your menu regularly to
    keep your meals

interesting and
nutritionally diverse.

Proactively addressing these common challenges, you can navigate the potential hurdles of adopting a whole-foods-based lifestyle with resilience and success. Remember that the journey is unique to each individual, and finding what works best for you is a key component of long-term adherence to a healthier way of eating.

CHAPTER 8

Incorporating Whole Foods into Your Lifestyle

Transitioning to a whole-foods-based lifestyle is a gradual process that involves mindful choices and considerations.

8.1 Gradual Integration

Adopting a whole-foods-based lifestyle doesn't have to happen overnight. Gradual integration allows for sustainable changes and makes the transition more manageable. Here's how to incorporate whole foods into your lifestyle gradually:

- **Start with Small Changes:**

  - Begin by making small changes to your meals. For example, incorporate an extra serving of vegetables into your dinner or swap a processed snack for a piece of fruit.

- **Focus on One Meal at a Time:**

  - Instead of revamping your entire diet, focus on one meal at a time. Start with breakfast, then move on to lunch, and finally, dinner. This step-by-step approach makes the process more achievable.

- **Experiment with New Ingredients:**

  - Explore unfamiliar whole foods and incorporate them into your meals. This could include trying a new vegetable, grain, or type of lean protein. Experimenting with different flavors keeps the process interesting.

- **Replace Processed with Whole:**

  - Gradually replace processed and refined foods with whole alternatives. For instance, choose whole grains instead of refined grains or opt for fresh fruit instead of sugary snacks.

- **Learn to Cook:**

  - Invest time in learning basic cooking skills. Cooking at home gives you control over the ingredients you use and allows you to experiment with whole foods in your own kitchen.

- **Listen to Your Body:**

  - Pay attention to how your body responds to changes. If you feel better and notice positive effects, it can serve as motivation to continue incorporating whole foods into your diet.

- **Set Realistic Goals:**

- Establish achievable
  goals for yourself. This
  could include committing
  to cooking at home a
  certain number of times
  per week or gradually
  reducing your intake of
  processed foods.

- **Celebrate Achievements:**

  - Celebrate your successes,
    no matter how small.
    Acknowledge the
    positive changes you've
    made and use them as
    motivation to continue
    your journey toward a
    whole-foods-based
    lifestyle.

8.2 Whole Foods on a Budget

Eating whole foods on a budget is possible with strategic planning and smart shopping. Here are tips for incorporating whole foods into your lifestyle without breaking the bank:

- **Buy in Bulk:**

  - Purchase staple items like grains, legumes, and nuts in bulk. This often comes at a lower cost per unit and reduces packaging waste.

- **Explore Frozen Produce:**

  - Frozen fruits and vegetables are often more affordable than fresh, and they have a longer shelf life. They can be just as nutritious and are convenient for quick meals.

- **Shop Seasonally:**

    - Purchase fruits and vegetables that are in season. Seasonal produce is not only fresher but also tends to be more budget-friendly.

- **Plan Meals and Use Leftovers:**

    - Plan your meals for the week, create a shopping list, and buy only what you need. Use leftovers creatively to minimize food waste.

- **Opt for Store Brands:**

- Consider trying store-
  brand products, as they
  are often more budget-
  friendly than name
  brands. Compare prices
  and nutritional
  information to make
  informed choices.

- **Explore Discount Stores and Farmers' Markets:**

  - Discount stores and
    farmers' markets can
    offer more affordable
    options for fresh produce
    and other whole foods.
    Compare prices and
    quality to find the best
    deals.

- **Buy in Season and Freeze:**

  - When certain fruits or
    vegetables are in season

and priced lower, consider buying in bulk and freezing for later use. This allows you to enjoy seasonal produce throughout the year.

- **Look for Sales and Discounts:**

  - Keep an eye out for sales, discounts, and promotions on whole foods. Buying items on sale can significantly reduce your grocery expenses.

- **Meal Prep and Cook at Home:**

  - Cooking at home is generally more cost-effective than dining out. Plan your meals, batch-cook when possible, and pack lunches to save money.

- **Consider Plant-Based Proteins:**

  - Plant-based protein sources like beans, lentils, and tofu are often more budget-friendly than some animal proteins. Integrate these into your meals for cost-effective and nutritious options.

Incorporating these gradual integration and budget-friendly tips, you can make the transition to a whole-foods-based lifestyle in a way that is sustainable, enjoyable, and economically viable. Remember that every positive change you make contributes to your overall well-being.

8.3 Sustainable Practices

Incorporating sustainable practices into your whole-foods-based lifestyle not only benefits your health but also contributes to the well-being of the planet. Here are tips for adopting sustainable practices along with your commitment to whole foods:

1. **Choose Local and Seasonal Produce:**

    - Opt for locally grown and seasonal fruits and vegetables. Supporting local farmers reduces the carbon footprint associated with transportation, and seasonal produce is often more flavorful and nutrient-dense.

2. **Reduce Food Waste:**

   - Plan meals, use leftovers creatively, and minimize food waste. Consider composting organic waste to further reduce your environmental impact.

3. **Use Reusable Bags and Containers:**

   - Bring reusable bags to the grocery store and use containers for bulk purchases to reduce single-use plastic waste. This simple change can have a significant impact on environmental sustainability.

4. **Minimize Packaging Waste:**

- Choose products with minimal packaging or those that use eco-friendly packaging. Buy in bulk when possible to reduce the overall amount of packaging.

5. **Explore Plant-Based Eating:**

   - Integrate more plant-based meals into your diet. Plant-based diets generally have a lower environmental footprint compared to diets high in animal products.

6. **Support Sustainable Fishing Practices:**

   - When choosing seafood, opt for sustainably sourced options. Look for certifications such as

MSC (Marine
Stewardship Council) to
ensure that the seafood
comes from responsibly
managed fisheries.

7. **Conserve Water:**

- Be mindful of water
  usage in food
  preparation. For
  example, use collected
  rainwater for watering
  plants and consider
  energy-efficient methods
  for cooking that use less
  water.

8. **Grow Your Own Food:**

- If possible, cultivate a
  small garden to grow
  your own herbs, fruits,
  and vegetables. This not
  only provides you with

fresh produce but also connects you to the process of food cultivation.

9. **Conscious Protein Choices:**

- Choose proteins that have a lower environmental impact. This includes plant-based proteins and those from sources with sustainable practices, such as grass-fed and pasture-raised options.

10. **Energy-Efficient Cooking:**

- Use energy-efficient appliances and practices in the kitchen. For example, cook with lids on pots to reduce cooking time, and choose

appliances with high
energy efficiency ratings.

11. Mindful Eating Habits:

- Practice mindful eating
to avoid
overconsumption. This
not only promotes better
digestion and enjoyment
of food but also reduces
the overall demand for
resources.

12. Educate Yourself and Others:

- Stay informed about
sustainable practices and
share your knowledge
with others. Awareness
and education contribute
to a broader movement
towards a more
sustainable food system.

13. **Consider Food Miles:**

- Be conscious of the distance your food travels to reach your plate. Choosing locally sourced options whenever possible reduces the environmental impact associated with transportation.

14. **Participate in Community Supported Agriculture (CSA):**

- Joining a CSA program allows you to receive fresh, locally grown produce directly from farmers. This supports local agriculture and helps build a sense of community.

15. **Reduce Red Meat Consumption:**

- Reducing the consumption of red meat, especially beef, can have a positive impact on both personal health and environmental sustainability. Consider incorporating more plant-based protein sources and lean meats.

Integrating these sustainable practices into your whole-foods-based lifestyle, you contribute to a healthier planet while enjoying the numerous benefits of a nutrient-rich diet. Remember, even small changes can make a meaningful difference over time.

CHAPTER 9

Tracking Progress

Monitoring your progress is an essential aspect of maintaining a whole-foods-based lifestyle.

9.1 Monitoring Health Changes

Regularly monitoring your health allows you to observe the positive impact of your whole-foods-based lifestyle. Here's how to track health changes:

- **Keep a Food Journal:**

    - Record your daily food intake, including meals, snacks, and beverages. Note how different foods make you feel and any changes in energy levels, digestion, or mood.

- **Check Physical Metrics:**

    - Track physical metrics such as weight, body measurements, and body fat percentage. Remember that changes may occur gradually, so be patient and consistent in your measurements.

- **Monitor Energy Levels:**

  - Pay attention to your energy levels throughout the day. Whole foods provide sustained energy, so you may notice improvements in energy stability and reduced energy crashes.

- **Assess Digestive Health:**

  - Observe changes in digestive health, including regularity, bloating, and discomfort. Increased fiber from whole foods often positively impacts digestive function.

- **Evaluate Sleep Quality:**

- Note any changes in sleep quality. Whole foods rich in certain nutrients, such as magnesium, can contribute to improved sleep patterns.

- **Track Mental Well-being:**

  - Monitor your mental well-being, including mood and cognitive function. Nutrient-dense foods can support brain health and positively influence mood.

- **Measure Fitness Progress:**

  - If you engage in physical activity, track improvements in fitness levels. This could include increased endurance,

strength, flexibility, or
any other fitness goals
you have set.

- **Regular Health Check-ups:**

  - Schedule regular health
    check-ups with
    healthcare professionals.
    Blood tests and other
    medical assessments can
    provide valuable insights
    into the impact of your
    dietary choices on key
    health indicators.

9.2 Celebrating Milestones

Celebrating milestones keeps you
motivated and reinforces the positive
changes you've made. Here's how to
celebrate your achievements along the
way:

- **Set Achievable Goals:**

    - Establish realistic short-term and long-term goals. Celebrate reaching these milestones, whether they involve weight loss, increased energy, or other health improvements.

- **Reward Yourself:**

    - Treat yourself to non-food rewards when you achieve a milestone. This could include a relaxing spa day, a new piece of workout gear, or any other reward that aligns with your preferences.

- **Share Successes with Others:**

- Share your achievements
    with friends, family, or a
    supportive community.
    Celebrating together
    creates a positive
    environment and
    reinforces your
    commitment to a whole-
    foods-based lifestyle.

- **Reflect on Progress:**

  - Take time to reflect on
    how far you've come.
    Acknowledge the
    positive changes you've
    made and the effort
    you've invested in
    improving your health.

- **Document Success Stories:**

  - Keep a journal of success
    stories or testimonials
    from others who have

embarked on a similar journey. Reading about others' successes can inspire and motivate you.

- **Create a Vision Board:**

  - Develop a vision board with visual representations of your goals. Display it in a prominent place as a daily reminder of the positive changes you're working towards.

9.3 Adjusting Your Approach

Flexibility and adaptability are key to long-term success. If needed, consider adjusting your approach to better suit your evolving needs:

- **Listen to Your Body:**

  - Pay attention to how your body responds to different foods and dietary patterns. If certain foods don't agree with you or if you experience changes in energy levels, consider adjustments.

- **Reassess Goals:**

  - Periodically reassess your goals to ensure they align with your current priorities and lifestyle. Adjust goals as needed, whether they involve nutrition, fitness, or overall well-being.

- **Seek Professional Guidance:**

- Consult with healthcare professionals, dietitians, or fitness experts if you encounter challenges or if you're unsure about aspects of your whole-foods-based lifestyle. Their expertise can provide valuable insights.

- **Experiment with New Recipes:**

  - Keep your meals exciting and satisfying by experimenting with new whole-foods-based recipes. This prevents monotony and helps you discover enjoyable and nutritious options.

- **Modify Exercise Routine:**

- If you engage in physical activity, consider modifying your exercise routine to keep it challenging and enjoyable. This could involve trying new activities, increasing intensity, or incorporating different types of workouts.

- **Adapt to Lifestyle Changes:**

  - Be adaptable to changes in your lifestyle, such as work commitments, travel, or family responsibilities. Modify your approach to ensure that your whole-foods-based lifestyle remains realistic and sustainable.

- **Stay Informed:**

  - Stay informed about nutrition and health trends. New research and insights may provide valuable information that can enhance your approach to a whole-foods-based lifestyle.

Regularly assessing and adjusting your approach allows you to tailor your whole-foods-based lifestyle to your individual needs and preferences. Remember that the journey is dynamic, and being open to adjustments ensures continued progress and success.